HOPE'S HOSPICE

AND OTHER POEMS

ALSO BY KWAME DAWES

POETRY
Resisting the Anomie (Goose Lane Editions)
Progeny of Air
Prophets
Jacko Jacobus
Requiem
Shook Foil
Mapmaker (Smith Doorstop chapbook)
Midland (Ohio University Press)
New and Selected Poems
Bruised Totems (Parallel Press chapbooks)
Wisteria Twilight Songs from the Swamp Country (Red Hen Press)
I Saw Your Face (children's poetry)
Brimming (Stepping Stone Press)
Gomer's Song (Black Goat)
Impossible Flying

ANTHOLOGIES
Wheel and Come Again: An Anthology of Reggae Poetry
Red (forthcoming)

FICTION
A Place to Hide
She's Gone (Akashic Books)
Bivouac (forthcoming)

NONFICTION
Natural Mysticism: Towards a New Reggae Aesthetic
Talk Yuh Talk: Interviews with Anglophone Caribbean Poets (University Press of Virginia)
Bob Marley: Lyrical Genius (Bobcat Press)
Twenty: South Carolina Poetry Fellows (Hub City Writers Project)
A Far Cry from Plymouth Rock: A Personal Narrative

Except where noted all titles above are published by Peepal Tree Press and available from www.peepaltreepress.com

HOPE'S HOSPICE

AND OTHER POEMS

KWAME DAWES

P E E P A L   T R E E

First published in Great Britain in 2009
Peepal Tree Press Ltd
17 King's Avenue
Leeds LS6 1QS
UK

ISBN 13: 9781845230784

Peepal Tree gratefully acknowledges Arts Council support

ACKNOWLEDGMENTS

These poems were written while I was on assignment in 2007 for the *Virginia Quarterly Review* reporting on HIV/AIDS in Jamaica. The project was sponsored by the Pulitzer Center On Crisis Reporting. Thanks to Jon Sawyer and Nathalie Applewhite for their commitment to this work, their persistence in promoting it, and for their encouragement. Thanks to Josh Cogan for his amazing photographs which are featured here. Thanks to the staff and crew of The Pulitzer Center for all the work that has gone into this project. Thanks also to the bluecadet web geniuses for their amazing website where these poems first appeared: www.livehopelove.com. Thanks to Kevin Simmonds who set many of these poems to music, and, in the process, helped me to see them afresh as I edited them for publication. Thanks to all the people who participated in this project, opening doors, arranging contacts, making time to share. Thanks to the people in Jamaica who told me their stories, took me into their private worlds and reminded me of the grace and resilience that blooms even in the most difficult of circumstances in Jamaica. This book is dedicated to my friends in Jamaica living with HIV/AIDS and the people who have been caring for them and spreading the word of tolerance and understanding about this disease. A special thanks and remembrance to the late John Mazourca of Hope Hospice in Montego Bay whose spirit humbles me still. Thanks to Jeremy and Hannah of Peepal Tree Press for their professionalism, friendship and sharp eyes. Thanks also to Charlene Spearen whose encouragement and tireless labours as a co-conspirator in poetry in South Carolina has played no small role in allowing me the space to write. Finally, thanks to my family, my children, and my wife Lorna for their support and permission.

See www.LiveHopeLove.com, an interactive web presentation that synthesizes audio and text versions of the poems, the Foreign Exchange videos, additional video interviews, music by Kevin Simmonds and photography by Joshua Cogan.
See www.vqronline.org/articles/2008/spring/dawes-aids-jamaica for Kwame Dawes's article 'Learning to Speak: The New Age of HIV/AIDS in the other Jamaica'.

for
Kojo, Aba, Adjoa, Gwyneth, Kojovi
for
Mama the Great
for
Sena, Kekeli and Akua
and for
Lorna for being there always
Remembering
Neville

CONTENTS

Hope's Hospice	9
Coffee Break	12
Nichol	13
Live Up	15
Making Ends Meet	16
Unforgiveness	19
Portmore	21
News	25
Fear	28
A Vanity	32
Yap	34
Lady Bee	36
Smile	38
Storm	40
Altar	43
Dance	47
Cleaning	48
Faith	50
Farm Work	54
Quilt	56
Sketch	61
Rainbow over Hope Road	64

HOPE'S HOSPICE
For John Mazourca

These days, the language of death
is a dialect of betrayals; the bodies
broken, placid as saints, hobble
along the tiled corridors, from room
to room. Below the dormitories
is a white squat bungalow, a chapel
from which the handclaps and choruses
rise and reach us like the scent
of a more innocent time.

I am trying to listen to the plump
Palestinian man with his swaying
rural middle-class patois, this jovial
servant, his eyes watering at the memory
of the eleven year old girl brought
to die inside these white walls,
her small body fading, her eyes
fierce with light and hungry
for wide open spaces, for decades
of discovery ahead of her.
When she came her mind was still
unable to calculate the treachery
of rape, to grasp how a man
could seek revenge on her tender body;
why as he wept when they took him
away, she wept, too, like the day
she wept when they took her mother's
empty body away, the disease
leaving her with nothing but bones,
thin skin, the scent of chickens.

I seek refuge in distractions:
the chapel of charms down the hill;
the pure sound of my youth,
when, cleansed by the perpetual blood,
my sins were never legion enough
for despair; when the comfort
of the Holy Spirit was green as this
sloping escarpment, thick with trees,
cool against the soft sunlight.

The plump man brushes
the gleam of tears from his cheeks.
I think of the simple equations
of compassion; I think of songs,
the harmonica, the strained
harmonies, the bodies of the dying
shuffling past, eyes still hoping;
the van waiting in the shade
to take me from all this;
the long ride through rain and dark
to Kingston, to sleep and more sleep.

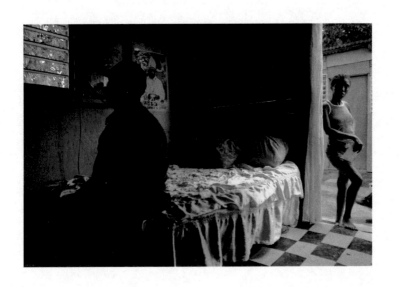

COFFEE BREAK

It was Christmas time,
the balloons needed blowing,
and so in the evening
we sat together to blow
balloons and tell jokes,
and the cool air off the hills
made me think of coffee,
so I said, "Coffee would be nice,"
and he said, "Yes, coffee
would be nice," and smiled
as his thin fingers pulled
the balloons from the plastic bags;
so I went for coffee,
and it takes a few minutes
to make the coffee
and I did not know
if he wanted cow's milk
or condensed milk,
and when I came out
to ask him, he was gone,
just like that, in the time
it took me to think,
cow's milk or condensed;
the balloons sat lightly
on his still lap.

NICHOL

How coolly it has broken you,
trying to mask the knowing
wit behind your eyes;

every smile, brilliant
against your gleaming
black skin, is defiance.

You stammer, push out
words, tell your story;
slap your knees to show

where your stroke-frozen
body would crawl
across the concrete

to reach the yard
with the gawking
onlookers. You laugh.

"Man must live.
Man must live."
How casually broken.

Tall lanky man,
hands clawed, yams
dangling, and the sweet

club man's charm
in your grin, still. All those
women slain by your art.

You stretch out your legs,
tell your story slow,
persistent as the crawl

you made towards sunlight,
the way you pulled
your body upright,

the way you made tender
the toughness of hard men
who would soon wash you,

feed you with oily fingers
full of mashed ackee
and tomatoes, who would

hold you against
the night, men, tough
as teeth, hard men.

"Man must live.
Man must live."
The virus prances

through your blood,
manages to tickle,
make you laugh

at a new sunny day –
and yours is the posture
of survival.

LIVE UP
For Nichol

How it had me
I couldn't talk.

This what you hear
is like water flow.

How it had me
I couldn't walk.

You might a call me cripple
but this cripple can walk.

How it had me
all I wanted to do

was crawl in a ball
and dead like that,

but see me here now,
see me here now,

man must live, iyah,
man must live.

MAKING ENDS MEET

She sells box juice every day
down by the terminus in Spanish
Town, to make ends meet, get
a little something for school
lunch and bus fare for her
big daughter whose body
is fine like hers, skinny
like breeze could blow her –
tall hair, high bottom, nice
shape. Sometimes it come
in like they are sisters
when they step their way
through the muddy pothole
and marl lanes of Portmore's
dry-back streets, and same way
the men are always asking
for a double mint slam
with two schoolers; and she
knows how to smile, kiss
her teeth and drag her big
daughter along. The girl
now wearing same short
frock and halter top
her mother wears, and mother
know it's a matter of time
before she start show belly,
though she warn her daily,
but girl is girl, and this Jamaica
is a rough place with man
who will lay wait you,
sweet talk you, offer you
bus fare and food money

each day, and sometimes
he might buy you a nice
shoes — just a matter of time.
And what a mother
who hustling a two cents
selling box juice and icy mint
down by the terminus
in her fade-out denim skirt
and broken down clog shoes,
with the fabric mangy down
to nothing where her tough
heel must rub every time
she step, can offer to this girl
who start to smell herself,
start to want things?
Fifty dollars for a bag a ice,
the rest is the heat and dust
of the city to make people
thirsty, make them buy.
Ever since she test positive,
nothing won't go right
for her; it come in like
a curse to blight her day —
big woman like this
depend on her mother
for clothes money
for some dollars to buy
pads and panty — what a life!
Man is like a curse on her,
with sweet mouth and lies;
man just take and take,
and all them leave is trouble;
man is like the grave to her,
she see them coming and run.

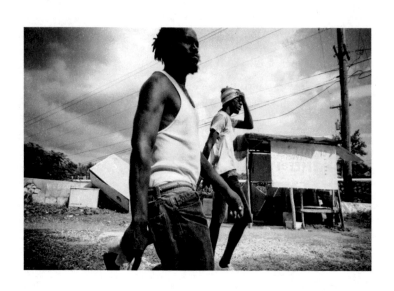

UNFORGIVENESS

"...while inside she knew the cold river was creeping up and up to extinguish that eye which must know by now that she knew..."

'Sweat' by Zora Neale Hurston.

1

Nothing like the surety of death
to make a skinny short man's
open hand seem like dust, an empty
weight on the skin. Look at him,
gabardine suit flopping about
his scrawny legs, loose shirt-tail
hanging, and the pride of chains,
rings, *chaparitas*. He is dying, too.
The same treachery in her blood
makes him as ordinary as dirt.

2

One year now since she gave up,
the stone in her belly
swelling into grotesquery –
a universe of errors. One year
now since the gurgle and greed
of his mouth pulling at anything
suckable. One year now since
the confession that his fainting,
his vomiting, his skin curdling
is AIDS in his blood. One year now
since she heard the news
of the end of her life – and now
no one speaks, no one has words
to offer her, no one can console.

Look at this short man,
ruler of his kingdom of worms,
reduced to this preening graveyard,
a man hustling some change
so he can eat from day to day,
a man who will sit and stare
into the sky, his eyes empty
of meaning, a man pleading
for her mercy while she eats
her daily meal in front of him —
a puppy begging for a morsel,
but she hisses her teeth,
leaves him snivelling.

She fears nothing now.
She laughs at his pathetic body
trying to rise with violence;
she laughs at how it crumbles
impotently. Once, at least, the fear
was part of the sweetness,
the assurance that something hard
was holding her. It's how death
simplifies things. It will take
us all; and she knows this well.
So her constant prayer is to live
long enough to see him plead
for his last sip of water.
She will take the glass brimming
with white light, and spill it
to the ground like libation
before his bewildered eyes.

PORTMORE

Here they turned swamp into marl pits,
stretches of reclaimed ground, fearing
always that storms would fill craters,
the tide rising to meet sudden stagnant
lakes, ruining the earth before it was ever glorious,
filling the air with drowsy mosquitoes.

Everything is flat here; acacia bushes
and dull green almond trees scattered along
the roadway squat like cowering crowds,
as if afraid to rise above it all, afraid of the slash
of the big machete; and at the city's gateway
stretches a line of bars and fish dens,
the stench of rotting fish and cooking
garbage thick over everything.

At dusk, the women line
the streets in red and garish green
and the quick flamboyant streak
of yellow; it is a basic trade – making
ends meet; holding body and soul
together; making dicks hard fast
to make them soft quick.

This is where Kingston has seeped
out new tribes that try to grow roots
in reluctant soil; the blood-letting continues
over the plains from the water's edge
to the scraggly heights of St Jago.

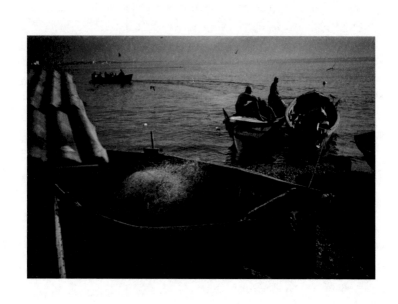

No palm trees here, not a coconut
frond in sight. We come to the crowded
beaches for the fish and festival
not for the water and black sand
in these grey foamy coves where
everything has died, and the fishermen
must push far out towards South America
to find a fresh fish to catch.

Here Lascelles, dressed in his green
gabardine suit, the well-pressed
olive shirt buttoned like a bad man
to the last button at the throat, struts
through this wilting city. Lascelles –
the man with a voice sweet as Delroy
Wilson, with the roots ruggedness
of soul-boy Dennis Brown, who could
dance bandy-legged like Ken Booth –
this small, sharp-headed man,
head up, strolls the side streets
with empty, useless hands, hoping that
now, since Labour is in, the green party
people will let him cut a tune,
capture a stage, burst like a hero
for that last triumph before the disease
in his blood, the disease that shadows
even the sound of his name, takes him.

Snap a shot of Lascelles leaning back
against a pink wall, shades over his eyes,
left foot pressed against the wall, hands
tucked deep into his pocket, with a cluster
of lazing women, conserving their energy,
waiting for a regular to come by for a quick

one. He sings into the night, his head
thrown back, his head swaying,
that voice carrying over the squalor,
making these women look up
for a moment, seeing for the first time
in a long time, the magic of an open sky.

NEWS

At first you look at your naked self
and you hold your dick in your hand,
and you think, "All this, all this
over some quick and fleeting fuck?"

Then you wait for it to stir, to let
you know it does not care
that it knows someone has lied,
but it remains silent, a dead thing.

You say you was minding your
business when the woman call
you, say you must come in,
take a test; you say you never know.

But people talk and you heard. Hannah
dead of AIDS. You remember
Hannah, her legs over your shoulder,
and the way she laughed, dear God!

Outside, you can't talk to a soul;
don't know where you must turn.
You want to take a shower, and shower
for days and days and days.

You lay your body out to rest.
People die everyday, so they say.
But this betrayal of desire
is a cruel, cruel thing, for true.

You think of all the pussies
you have plowed into bare back,
riding deep, trying to find that last
dying place. You think of corpses.

At dawn the street smells of gunpowder;
you have forgotten the fear of death;
you are reckless as the condemned;
hymns make you weep and tremble.

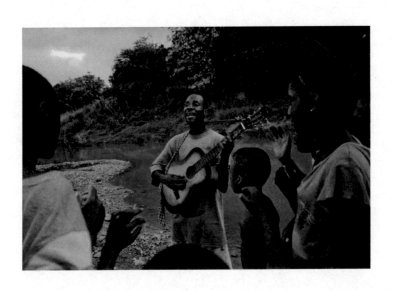

FEAR

1

No one will admit it, but this thing
that poems can't name, and songs can't

turn to metaphor, is as unreliable
as myth. Best to think of it as fear

or faith – the substance of things
to come; the evidence of things

we do not long for. Big John
Mazourca, the Palestinian shopkeeper,

knows all about faith in this thing –
the dead pile up. After this one

is taken away, the nun must guard
his things – the open-bellied transistor,

the stick deodorant, the toothpaste,
five hundred dollars, a paper bag

with a loaf of sweet bun, flip-flops
and the tattered pile of clothes –

she must guard them for days
until she is sure the family won't

come for its inheritance. Then
she parcels out the remains,

a judge, hearing the claims
of friendships and promises made.

It is something of a wake;
the transistor has survived

so many of these. John gathers
the soiled linens, washes them with

heavy-duty bleach, and hangs
them out to dry, a choreography

of pastels whooping in the breeze.
He finds comfort in the sweet green

of freshly mown grass. Then he gathers
the sun-warm sheets, stretches

them over the mattress, and waits
for the new one to come, eyes

still alert, as if faith has not
quite settled in.

2

What we don't say is that we don't
know what a rash looks like –
except we do, and this is the dilemma,

the mystery of miracles. And how
many blisters in a mouth does
it take to know? It takes faith

to read the constant yeasting
of a vagina as the answer
we have longed to know.

3

Take Paul —
long-faced, smooth-talking, sly
man — now he is a man of faith.

Fourteen years, he says, fourteen
years since they said the virus
was swimming in him, and he has lived

without a pill, just good food,
exercise and decent living,
though he doesn't know why,

but he believes what they say;
he has lived each day waiting
for the thing to turn to death in him.

He has forgotten the danger
of rushing traffic, the jujitsu
of cancer, the fear of drowning.

4

So, except for the unsaid things –
the lean and hungry look he sports,

the fourteen-year-old cough,
the night sweats, the flight of lovers,

the swelling brain – we say it is faith
like a mustard seed to believe this.

What we won't say is that we don't know,
and we won't know for certain until

the ravaging is upon us, and all fat is consumed,
and our cheeks collapse, and our skins curdle

with sores, and our lungs grow thick
with blood and phlegm, and we shit and shit

until there is nothing left to shit, and the glory
of our reckoning arrives. Until then, we carry

fear like a talisman of our hope,
our only evidence of what is to come.

A VANITY

O that this too too sullied flesh should melt,
Thaw and resolve itself into a dew....
William Shakespeare

I promise myself simple things –
like to fight to the death for my vanity,
to always chase after the damned wind,
for to live fully immersed in one's vanities
is surely to live. So I promise that Rachel Eliza
will bring her satchel of cameras and film
and drive me to an open field between
two mountains near a cottage
with its sky-blue walls,
when I have reached perfection, when
I have been sculpted down to one-eighty-
six pounds, and my hair has been trimmed
to a dark gleam over my skull,
and the veins in my arms are coiled
beautifully over the last breaths of muscle
before my bones take over.
For two weeks of elegance, I will
gambol and cavort shirtless and lewd,
offer my flat-bellied profile revealing
at last the ribs I lost so long,
and my navel will be a tight knot,
jutting slightly after being so long
in the dark well of my stomach.
In that sweet interim, I will be
as beautiful as I have dreamed to be,
and everyone will adore the shape
of my splendid emaciation – all this
before the joints bore against

my worn-out skin, before I join
the bone-yard of the walking dead.
It is the one promise I make
to myself, and it must happen in May
when the poui trees begin to yellow
and blue, and the world is in glorious
riot, and in that moment, everything
will be right with me, I promise.

YAP

He was remembered
his name becoming a common
noun and verb in regular parlance:

A yap

(/yap/ *n*. **yap yappist** /ya-pest/*vi* **yap yapped** /yap-t/ [Youthful
innovation Jamaica College] (1974) 1: HOMOSEXUAL usually
considered obscene; 2: battyman and specialist in homosexual
practices; 3: the scourge of school boys; 4: their secret fear when
clandestine hands cause self-inflicted sticky orgasms; 5: something
no boy admits he is to other boys. (*No longer in common usage*)

A gentle boy with a sharp tongue,
he played chess quickly, aggressively
winning with a laugh – played football

in a torn yellow shirt and red shorts;
his father sold radios and calculators
in an air-conditioned appliance store

somewhere downtown and made good money.
They lured him into the piss-stink toilet
flooded with piss and loose shit,

its blue walls scarred with obscenities –
secrets about teachers, yearnings,
hieroglyphics of a twisted culture.

Nunez, the short Syrian, was the bait
with his tight pants and benign smile –
securing his heterosexual credentials

despite his lisp and delicate eyes.
And they lured Yap into the toilet
where he thought he'd find a friend.

They beat his head till blood
washed the wet cement floor
and his blue shirt turned purple.

This dizzy day of crows circling,
heating to a haze the old cream buildings,
lonely on the feet-worn dust

under the tamarind tree
sat Yap, wiping the blood
from his broken teeth,

tears streaming, frantic to find words
to explain why he wanted to leave
this school and why his shirt was wet

like that. The Citroen sailed in
and stopped. The door opened, swallowed
Yap. The Citroen sailed out.

LADY BEE

Lady Bee is dead — that disease devoured him.
He lasted almost a year, then he died. Perhaps
the ribbons of tongues burst on his lips, aflame
in the ward. He broke into tongues like that
on the parade ground, his prayers in the midst
of the most ordinary acts. I did not know then
that it was his prayer-language, the tongue
of prophecy, the Holy Ghost in his heart
that took him when he least expected it: Love.

He is dead now, the Captain, the lanky
officer who sprinted brilliantly, but like a girl,
a strong, elemental girl who leaned and wind-
milled his arms on the turns before the eighty
yards home — perhaps negotiating the physics
of the Lord's voice in his head. Captain was
kind, a good guy, but he could not have
heard the Spirit that night when I found you,
and you whispered to me with your eyes —
so full of stones, questions, answers,
dreams, mysteries, shocks — that you could
fly, that you could read my mind, that you
could fly. No tongues hurled forward so I would
know what they had done to you — no Spirit
spoke. Everyone — Captain, too — was dumb.
Captain was Lieutenant then, then he climbed
to Captain, and later Major — I call him *Captain* still,
it suits him, how I trusted him then, captain, my captain.

He kept climbing. The Lord prospered him
in this world of miniature achievement,
while you stayed buck-private. Of course

you had your triumphs: you flew and sometimes tongues
would flare from you and we all looked around
for someone to translate – though no one did, not then,
not a single soul spoke, not friends,
not the good captain in his Sam Browns
and burnished boots, with his swanky
salute and clipped eyes-rights.

Today, you carry the news of the captain's passing.
Lady Bee is dead, you say with sadness; you tell me
it is a good thing he was ready – that they say he
spoke in tongues before his eyes rolled back
in reverie. I think of you as a saint, now;
the way you announce his end with love.

SMILE

But I am alive,
counting days,
holding up.

I have these pills
that make the fat
grow on my hips.

I have more ass
than I ever had,
making me roll

like any woman
dancing her way
through Edgewater.

If you tickle me,
I will laugh like
yesterday's child,

bellyful of heaven
and earth;
but come night –

all clichés persist –
I cry myself
to sleep asking

why? As if somewhere
in my dreams
someone will whisper

that there's been
a mistake,
that *positive*

is good
and *negative* is bad,
that my baby-father

is alive and dancing
against the sea's blue.
Come morning,

my face aches;
I break apart
my lips, and smile.

STORM

Kingston settles on your skin,
the grit of wood-fire and exhaust
on your body; you know sin,
the pleasure of untrammelled lust.

Kingston is green in November,
so much rain; the water runs
on the surface. I remember
the taste of fat June plums.

Most of my friends are dying –
it is their precious secret,
and the others are busy nursing
the dying. God's cruel edits.

I stand in this storm,
let its battering break me;
I know now every form
of death; no more mystery here.

The eye passes mutely;
and while the earth vomits,
and shingles cartwheel
around me, I doubt it

all: the conspiracy of death.
I will live to see the wasting
of my flesh; my last breath
will be in a calm season.

I will know my sins,
every betrayal; those I killed,
whose voices whisper in
my restless brain until

tears come, until praying
I slip away like night,
a frail man limping
towards morning light.

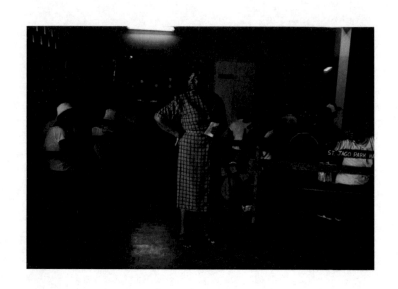

ALTAR
For Annesha

Mama settles in the shadows,
her prayers slip through the white

burglar bars, dance above the flat
concrete roofs, then dally over

Arnette Gardens where the stink
of a rotting dog in the drying gully,

mingles with the sweet comfort
of burning weed and jerking meat –

the pepper, the pimento, the molasses.
And she is praying hard-hard

that God will fly off the Blue Mountains,
travel down Marcus Garvey Drive,

turn into one of those ragged lanes
to this place they call a ghetto.

People just don't know
the many havens you can find here,

like this one where Mama kneels under
the shelter of crotons, aloe-vera,

hibiscus, and garish rose bushes;
where she has built an altar of gleaming

bleached rum bottles that stand
in a circle on a cruciform

platform, raised above the earth,
and in the middle an enamel pan is full

with water caught in the last rains
and strewn with petals.

At this shrine, Mama's voice
carries high above the news.

The voices are whispering to me:
Father Holung coming for you,

baby girl. Is your time now;
the priest in white with flaxen hair

coming for you. Your time now.
Pay them no mind, she says.

But they carry on through the night,
and before dawn, I prepare

my cocktail of Baygon and rum;
my cocktail of bleach and tar;

my cleansing, my purging,
my fire into this worthless body –

"AIDS a go kill me; AIDS a go
kill me." Poor Mama, how tiny

her voice sounds wailing for mercy;
asking God how come, how come;

and me praying for my daughters;
mercy, mercy until the shadow comes.

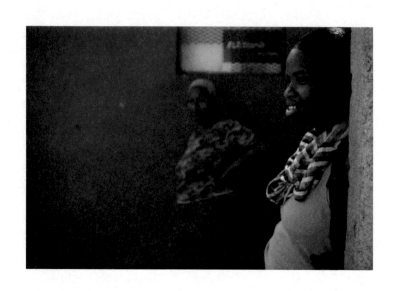

DANCE

Beenie Man in a white fedora
is legs all legs as he strides
like a king across the stage,
head held back, mic to mouth,
scatter-shot lyrics, gruff
as any bedroom-bully – and a girl
can forget her worries,
can blank out the belly's
groaning, can feel like
a girl child again, not no
baby mother thrice over
with no answers for tomorrow;
can silence the whisper
of the disease in her blood,
loose up her waistline,
and dance away the gloom;
Lord, dance inside the boom
of the sound system; dance
with this long, magga
black man in his white
tux commanding all
and sundry to roll
their bellies – and what else
to do but dance, baby,
sweat it out, find back
the sweet spot in the spine;
feel clean again,
feel fresh again, feel
rude again – while the city
shimmers with its
million souls trying
to make all sorrow
fade away, sweet Lord?

CLEANING

After a while, you don't bother
with the brief and the pajamas;
you leave him on the sheet,
make him shit himself,

then you shift him over
to the other side
until you can come, lift up
the body, wipe his bottom
with a soft cotton cloth,

bundle up the sheet
with the other two resting
in the corner, straighten
out the plastic over the mattress –

sometimes you have to wipe
it, too – then put a towel
under him until the other
sheet dry, and all the time,

you don't say a word,
you don't ask for nothing;
you let your hand brush
against your father's back

and pray his dignity will last
another day. This is how
a man must care for his father;
quiet, casual, and steady.

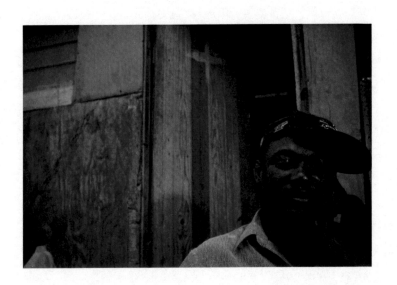

FAITH

for Nichol, Lorraine, Sherese, Lascelles, Glendon, Tricia, Renesha, Dave, Anneshia and Paul.

Now faith is the substance of things hoped for
The evidence of things not seen.
Hebrews 11:1

1
The Seen Things

The news comes like a stone falling.
Suddenly all light is gone.
Outside the heat is black as loss.
Tomorrow is a burden.
I speak the words into the air;
no one answers; the sky
is a dull plate of silences.
Tomorrow is a heavy load.
My feet move sluggishly,
every sound muted to a drone.
It is hard to dream these days,
and oh, the tears, the tears.

This treachery of the blood
is a secret rushing through me
and my face is a mask;
no one must read beyond
its inscrutable dumbness,
no one must know.

I cannot read the faces around me;
everyone seems filled with hope –
how pleasantly ordinary this life
must be for them, I think.
But who can read the secrets we carry
in this city of dust, exhaust
and the clamour of engines?

2
The Unseen Things

Hope is in the tender hands that hold you.
Hope is in the embrace of the loving.
Hope is in the flesh touching flesh
to remind us of our human selves.
Hope is in the gentle nod of recognition,
hope is in the limping body still pushing
against the pain, the discomfort, still
laughing from so deep down it feels
like the rush of alcohol in the head,
the full abandonment of all fear.
Hope is in the freedom to say
I long to feel the rush of desire
satisfied; hope is to embrace hunger
and find comfort in the sharing of needs.
Hope is in the hands we grasp,
the prayers we whisper,
the amen, the amen, the amen.

Evidence and Substance

There is substance in the gathering
of bodies battered by this disease.

There is evidence in the quiet promise
we make to be here again next week.

There is substance in the sweet taste
of coconut water, the scent of morning.

There is evidence in the songs a slim man
sings, healing as the balm of warmed oil.

There is substance in the expletives shattering
our peace, the tears, the lament, the fear.

There is evidence in the hum of recognition,
the comfort of hands held tightly.

There is substance in the streets walked
to tell people to hope for tomorrow.

There is evidence in the body growing fat
with love, round with hopefulness.

There is substance in the promises we make
to protect this world with the truth of our wounds.

There is evidence in the rituals of the living,
the memories of the lived, the calm we crave.

There is substance in the green of rainy season,
in the harvest of sweet mangoes in November.

There is evidence in these songs we now sing
against the treachery of our blood.

FARM WORK

Wouldn't guess *farrin* could be hot
like the worst heat on the Frome Estate;
even worse, the way you can't find
a tree as far as you look, and when you find
a *magga* piece of bush, and squat
your wet self in its shadow, you can't feel
even a breeze to ease things.

These days, the age is showing;
the body can't manage this work
no more; half a day and it come in
like I been working for a week
with not a break, not a sip of water;
and I know all I need is some *cerese* tea
and a good *senna* purge; all I need is anointing
oil and Mother Martha hand over me
to ease back this thing eating out my bones.

Last night the barracks start to smell of death –
a sweet nasty smell in my nose –
and no matter how much rum I knock back,
my mind travelling and the body trembling,
that sweet smell won't go away.
I don't eat a good meal in two weeks
and everything falling off my body.

This *farrin* is a bitch; not one kindness,
except for the belly of that Icilda
who set up shop here three years now
to make a lickle money, but mostly
she know how yard man need love,
need to hear a woman talk sweet

in a voice singing music they know;
and if it wasn't for she, I couldn't stand
to stay so long, couldn't take it.

Christmas coming and the dry town
stay same as always – the time
don't move – and I buying a little
something to carry with me.
Find a nice tie for the big boy
that will make him give up the Rasta
foolishness; a shoes for the girl –
she say she wanted red, but red
is for *tegareg* so I buy her blue;
and see this nice frock I buy
for the wife? She can wear red,
for she is my *tegareg*, my blessing.

But this sickness eating me up,
and I taking a stone in my hand
for tomorrow. I want to find a place
to rest my head again, a soft
belly to ease back on, and the cool green
light of my country where people know
my father's name, where a man can be man
among men, where God is in heaven
behind the Blue Mountains
and his voice ride over the trees
to reach my soul: that is home.

QUILT

1

Powell

In the belly of this postcard city
a brown stench covers everything –
the ripeness of open sewers, the sweaty

narrow lanes, the horde of mumbling
people, the seediness of tourists' pleasures;
it is this dark earth and grime

that gave us the broken treasure
of a man, this sufferer counting time –
each hour – before the sickness dragged

him down. He taught us in the trick
of his smile the way to heal. This bag
of bones, this counterpoint to the tragic,

this was Powell, a brother whose passing
stung us like sea salt in the wind.

2
Margaret

Margaret, your mother gave you this yellow
name when the light was just right

and there was music slowly blowing
through the open louvres. While your bright

eyes drank her in, she fed you milk
and a future of loss, before she withered

away, before she grew slowly sick,
before she died. Margaret, did you remember

the name she gave you when her man
plowed into your infant womb the curse

in his blood, when he crammed
into your tender self, his anger and terror?

How can you now smile, little girl, how do you
carry this burden as if it's a wisp of dew?

3

Mango

Thanks for your appetite for ripe mangoes.
I washed them in caught rain water, wiping
them down, then cutting them into two
succulent cups. Thank you for the eating,

your mouth moving quickly, your body
savouring every sting of Bombay sweetsour;
thank you for gleefully sucking each seed
till it was white; thank you for the heat

on your gleaming head; the gurgling melody
of your pleasure; thank you that though
you became sick, yet you thanked me
for my gift to you. I pray that tomorrow

you will wake in mango heaven, feasting
on bushels of sweet, your renewed body shining.

4
Leaving

I would have wanted you to live longer,
but your healing came as forgiveness,
to doubt which would be to remember
the vomit you can't return to. The rest
of my days will be filled with me
trying not to forget, searching for a clue
of you in every ordinary thing – ackee trees,
a freshly picked June plum, the startling blue
of a three o'clock sky. I am still annoyed
with God for offering the lie of healing,
but he must know how to call his own
in his own peculiar way. All this leaving
is too much for me. You should have stayed,
my dear friend, that's all I know to say.

5

Quilt

Eventually, the expanding quilt grew too long
for the hall wall, and the stitching,

so hurriedly done, was no longer strong
enough to hold the fabric; the fading

initials fell limp, and folks were missing
their names. Five went last week, with no one

cutting strips of cloth, no one gathering
to hum prayers – they were just gone. Dying

has become ordinary and reminders are too much.
So we've moved the quilt to the store room,

folded it into a simple box. On the porch,
three simple candles burn, the gloom

of dusk broken by the vigil of flames;
in the trees' whisper you hear their names.

SKETCH

With graphite I soften your bones,
make exotic the absence of your lashes,
show your fingers, long and elegant,
cradling a plum, the light of its juice
flaming vermillion through the taut skin.

I etch out your gaze, tender, tender
about your forehead where the pain
has seared the skin, softly
as if, in the soft lead, I can calm
it all, make it go away. You are going.

With the soft of my palm's heel
I caress the bald glow of your head,
then clean a grey line where your brows
were – now there is nothing –
these markings of what you have suffered.

These days, bodies crumble
about me, the dead, desperate for healing,
grow weary, stoic, then quietly go.

My blackened fingers make you round,
plump as a fruit just plucked.
Tomorrow I lift you, bird of bones,
limbs softly collapsed.

There is sunlight crawling across the lawn.
Despite the drought, it's resiliently green,
except the narrow path of old sod we laid,
now traumatized by neglect into a crude buzz-cut;
and this, too, tells us what we have lost.

It is August in Kingston. Nothing can fight in this heat. Just stay still, maybe a small wind will blow, maybe a small wind.

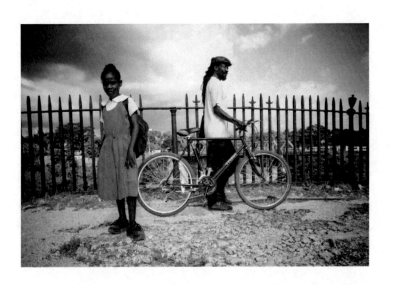

RAINBOW OVER HOPE ROAD

And for just that instant,
when from Hope Road

we watched the rainbow cut
across the robust body

of the Blue Mountains,
the way the sun seemed

filtered and clean
as peace, when the gleam

of quick colour bounced
giddily off the cars,

we offered quiet gratitude
for fleeting lasting things.

BIOGRAPHIES

Born in Ghana in 1962, **Kwame Dawes** spent most of his childhood and early adult life in Jamaica. As a poet, he is profoundly influenced by its rhythms and textures, citing in a recent interview his "spiritual, intellectual, and emotional engagement with reggae music." His book, *Natural Mysticism*, explores that engagement.

He has published fifteen collections of poetry, a poetry anthology, two works of fiction, four works of non-fiction and a play. His essays have appeared in numerous journals including *Bomb Magazine*, *The London Review of Books*, *Granta*, *Essence*, *World Literature Today* and *Double Take Magazine*.

Future publications include new collections of poetry, *Back of Mount Peace* and *Wheels*, a poetry anthology, *Red*, and *Bivouac*, a novel.

Kwame Dawes is Distinguished Poet in Residence, Louis Frye Scudder Professor of Liberal Arts and Founder and executive Director of the South Carolina Poetry Initiative. He is the director of the University of South Carolina Arts Institute and the programming director of the annual Jamaican Calabash International Literary Festival. He is the associate poetry editor at Peepal Tree Press.

Joshua Cogan writes:
"After graduating with a Masters degree in anthropology, I ditched the ivory tower and took to the road with a mission to document vanishing cultures through photography and new media. My personal work revolves heavily around faith and culture, and environment and culture. I've produced a number of innovative projects with the award-winning multimedia firm Blue Cadet, including the study of how high school students displaced by Hurricane Katrina have coped with the loss of a way of life."

He lives in Washington D.C. and his work has appeared in *The New Yorker*, the *Washington Post*, *New York Times*, *GQ* and *Men's Health*. His work can be seen at www.joshuacogan.com and at www.livehopelove.com.

NEW POETRY FROM PEEPAL TREE PRESS
Spring-Summer 2009

Marion Bethel
Bougainvillea Ringplay
ISBN: 9781845230845; pp. 88, July 2009; £7.99

These poems are sensual in the most literal sense – the poems are about the senses, the smell of vanilla and sex, the sound of waves – radio, voices, sea; the taste of crab soup; the texture of hurricane wind, and the chaos of colours bombarding the eye. Bahamian poetry is being defined in the work of Marion Bethel.

Jacqueline Bishop
Snapshots from Istanbul
ISBN: 9781845231149; pp. 80, April 2009; £7.99

Framed by poems that explore the lives of the exiled Roman poet Ovid, and the journeying painter Gaugin, Bishop locates her own explorations of where home might be. This is tested in a sequence of sensuous poems about a doomed relationship in Istanbul, touching in its honesty and, though vivid in its portrayal of otherness, highly aware that the poems' true subject is the uprooted self.

Frances Marie Coke
Intersections
ISBN: 9781845230845; pp. 106, August 2009; £7.99

Francis Coke writes with eloquent empathy and profound insight about the difficult truths of family relations, abandonment, loneliness, and the challenges of faith when hope is hard to find. She writes about Jamaica's poverty, violence, class divides and racial complexities with the same tenderness that she writes about its people.

Mahadai Das
A Leaf in His Ear
ISBN: 978900715591; pp. 160, May 2009; £9.99

The selection includes the whole of *Bones* and *My Finer Steel Will Grow*, and most of the poems from her first collection, *I Want to Be a Poetess of My People*, as well as many of the fine poems published in journals and previously uncollected – from lively, humorous nation-language poems to the oblique, highly original poems written in the years after *Bones*.

Millicent A.A. Graham
The Damp in Things
ISBN: 9781845230838; pp. 56, May 2009; £7.99

In *The Damp in Things*, we are invited into the unique imagination of Millicent Graham: she offers us a way to see her distinctly contemporary and urban Jamaica through the slant eye of a surrealist, one willing to see the absurdities and contradictions inherent in its society. These are poems about family, love, spirituality, fear, and above all desire, where the dampness of things is as much about the humid sensuality of this woman's island as it is about her constant belief in fecundity, fertility and the unruliness of the imagination.

Esther Phillips
The Stone Gatherer
ISBN: 9781845230852; pp. 72, May 2009; £7.99

Tracing a woman-centred movement from childhood to the contemplative maturity of elder and prophet, Esther Phillips's affecting new collection is the work of a poet of wit, intelligence, and maturity of vision. She uses poetry to test the meaning of experience, and to seek and find its grace notes. Located in the moving, breathing landscape of Barbados, and displaying a lyrical West Indian English, this collection marks her as a major poetic voice.

Jennifer Rahim
Approaching Sabbaths
ISBN: 9781845231156; pp. 129, July 2009; £8.99

There is a near perfect balance between the disciplined craft of the poems, and their capacity to deal with the most traumatic of experiences in a cool, reflective way. Equally, she has the capacity to make of the ordinary something special and memorable. The threat and reality of fragmentation – of psyches, of lives, of a nation – is ever present, but the shape and order of the poems provide a saving frame of wholeness.

Tanya Shirley
She Who Sleeps with Bones
ISBN: 9781845230876; pp. 76, April 2009; £7.99

'In the deftly searching poems of *She Who Sleeps With Bones*, Tanya Shirley considers how memory revolts from oblivion, what it can mean to be "haunted by the fruit" of desire – sexual, political, the desire for an "uncomplicated legacy," for home when home exists only as a memory we cannot trust entirely, a space we fear even as we continue to go back there. These poems startle, stir, provoke equally with their intelligence and their music. A wonderful debut.'

— Elizabeth Nunez, author of *Prospero's Daughter*